NUTRITION AND
WEIGHT CONTROL
SIMPLIFIED

NUTRITION AND
WEIGHT CONTROL
SIMPLIFIED

John Batchelor

To order additional copies of this book, contact:
Xlibris LLC
1-888-795-4274
www.Xlibris.com
Orders@Xlibris.com
663180

NUTRITION AND WEIGHT CONTROL SIMPLIFIED—PART ONE

We are born with some human instincts, but we have no real knowledge of what this crazy world of ours is all about, so we have to turn to our parents for some primary knowledge and this may be knowledgeable or it may just be very uninformed and apathetic.

They obtained their knowledge from their parents and others, depending on their circumstances and may have given it a lot of thought or none at all.

At any rate that is all we have available at this time and as we grow older, we come in contact with others that may have an effect on what we believe.

If we are smart, we will not just accept anything that others tell us and give it some serious thought of our own, but try not to just reject everything that is different to what we have been taught either the smartest person in the world doesn't know everything and the dumbest knows things that we don't know, so listen to everybody and then make your own decisions.

The responsibility for your health lies with you.

Nutrition is only one of these things and what I am interested in for the moment.

Parents are usually not a big help and have already developed their own bad habits.

Most likely they are the ones that introduced you to junk food, because they were already hooked on it.

Even if they didn't, the parents of your friends may have influenced them and they in turn influence you.

When I was a kid there wasn't the preponderance of junk food as there is today, but I didn't get much anyway as my parents had survived tougher times and were very frugal and didn't want to spend money on it, but at home, my mother cooked with more thought to what food tasted like than what was good for our health and I think most people do the same. She used a lot of sugar and butter in her dishes and although I had eggs for breakfast once in a while, more likely I had a bowl of Rice Krispies, loaded with sugar and whole milk and peanut butter sandwiches with jelly on white bread, a baloney sandwich on white bread or a grilled cheese sandwich on white bread and slathered with butter was a standard lunch for me and most likely one sandwich was not enough for my young appetite.

I don't remember ever hearing the word snack, it was not even in my vocabulary.

Lemonade, loaded with sugar was considered something worthy to drink, because it was tasty and refreshing on a hot day.

Supper was always some kind of meat fried in bacon grease that my mother saved on top of the stove in a tin can or some crisco lard and many times breaded with white refined flour, a can of veggies, warmed up with a chunk of butter and a half cup of sugar added and usually a glass or two of sweet tea.

When she had time, she would make brownies, fudge, pies and cakes and by ten years old, she taught me to make them as well. She had the original Betty Crockers cookbook that she swore by.

Even though I didn't get much that was considered "Junk food", I developed type 2 diabetes and my mother died from it at an early age.

Since then many people write cookbooks and have TV shows teaching others how to cook in this unhealthy and irresponsible manner and get paid for it.

The power of suggestion is a powerful influence in our lives, but just like everything else, we need to learn to think for ourselves, when possible and not just be a sheep herded into pasture.

I have always been interested in my health, but had no clear idea of what that was. I would hear a little something from whomever and just accept that as fact.

Years ago, doctors did not even routinely check our blood for Glucose and cholesterol levels,etc. and I have yet to meet a doctor that knows much about nutrition or at least has told me what is what, they are what I call "Bandaid doctors" with little to no thought about prevention. "Pill pushers" may be an even better nickname for them.

"You need to lose some weight!" "Can you tell me how?" "Yes, don't eat so much!" Even those that claim to be experts constantly contradict each other confusing us.

To make matters more confusing, we are bombarded with people trying to sell us "Magic bullets", pretending to have our health interests at heart. Buried in this barrage of nonsense is some nuggets of truth and it is left for us to find them and pull them out of the trash.

Most of us, being busy working, raising families and trying to find ways to enjoy our life, have just picked at our nutritional needs, while those that would fleece us out of our money, keep us rushing back and forth, chasing an easy fix to our health, wasting our time, money and health as well. There is a barrage of books out there now and many have a little good information, buried in with some not so good or incomplete information and some are just downright stupid and irresponsible.

I have no credentials to offer and don't claim to be an expert on anything, but I have spent the last few years after my retirement devoted to trying to sort out this mess and have wasted a lot of money chasing rainbows and reading many books, pulling my hair out and doing experiments of my own and giving it a lot of thought and this essay is just about what I believe and what I do and you can decide for yourself if you think I am correct, partially correct or just full of you know what.

There are some things that we know are false and some things that are undisputed, making them possibly true.

Here is my take -

Just like everything else, beware of those that endeavor to sell you something. They may be legit, but unfortunately, buried in the surrounding nonsense. Its like trying to find a needle in a haystack. When things sound too good to be true, they usually are.

Never forget the old saying "Caveat emptor" "let the buyer beware!" (This doesn't just pertain to nutrition)

When tiny pills are supposed to help you lose weight or improve your nutrition, they may contain a teensy, weensy bit of beneficial ingredients, but not enough to have any real effects, except the placebo effect that you may have attached to them, wanting them to work and some are downright detrimental to your health. They are certainly not worth throwing good money away on them to find out, like I and so many other people have already done, So...............

Nowadays there are more and more people becoming interested in their health and probably already know what foods are obviously not good for our health and just maybe what is good.

Unfortunately I find that most people are just interested in their weight and not in their overall health. Certainly, being over or underweight is not healthy, but it is far from the whole story.

Counting calories, while ignoring the nutritional value is fallacy and not in your bodys best interest.

Eating in a nutritionally acceptable way will not cure every ailment, but will certainly give your body the best chance to help itself prevent and maybe even cure some of the issues.

Lets explore and give this a lot of thought together and see what we come up with. Keep in mind that variety is not only the spice of life, it is essential for optimum health. No two foods bring the exact same nutritional value to the table and moderation is the name of the game.

Just because one food is rated superior to others doesn't mean to not eat a variety of the others. Strawberries for instance are rated nutritionally higher than any other fruit and three times higher than blueberries, but blueberries bring their own special benefits to our diet, just like every other food does. Overeating a couple of foods, no matter the nutritional value, will not do. Spinach is rated much higher than any other food, but is also rated the highest in Oxalates, which may be detrimental to your health if overeaten. Popeye was on the right track, but he didn't have all the information needed for good decisions.

You could even die if you drink too much water at one time. (I dont want to scare you, it would take an awful lot and is extremely rare, but I just wanted to make a point)

Moderation, variety and proper combinations of food is the answer.

CALORIES

Protein has 4 calories per gram
carbohydrates have 4 calories per gram
fat has 9 calories per gram

At any rate that is the accepted statistics. I have some doubts about the accuracy of this information, but it doesn't really matter, its still offers the best information that we have to go on.

GLYCEMIC INDEX

This is the amount that a given food or combination of food will drive up your blood sugar, but it is difficult to find any reliable information on it. The little that I have found from different sources, contradict each other, so.........This is known as blood Glucose spiking and we will soon learn a little more about it.

HUMANS

A few have superior brain power than the rest of us and to other animals, but in many ways other animals are superior. They usually have better eyesight, are stronger, faster, etc, crocodiles can manufacture their own teeth replacements for their whole life, without ever seeing a dentist. They instinctively know what food they should be eating. Only humans kill for fun, greediness and just because somebody else doesn't look like us or have the same thoughts.

Maybe we can't do a lot about what other people do, but we are the Captains of our own ships and can do a lot to improve ourselves and taking care of our health to the best of our ability is one of the most important.

JUNK FOOD

This is a huge money maker and no one that manufacturers them or sells them gives any thought to your health, only to their pocketbook. I don't even know what most of these things are and some that I have tasted are disgusting to me, but apparently others have a different set of taste buds, but I do like the taste of a few of them and they can become addictive or at least a bad habit, but just try to avoid them as much as possible.

You know what they are. If you don't feel that you are capable of giving them up at least learn to make better choices and try to cut down on all of them as much as possible, without losing your sanity.

If you are diabetic you have special incentive to avoid foods that drive up your blood glucose levels too much and this doesn't just go for junk food, but even healthy food as well. Potato chips are considered by some to be the worst thing you could possibly eat. A very thin slice of nutritious potato, but high in glycemic index and calories, saturated with oil that we don't really know what it is and tons of salt and what is little heard about, is added sugar and don't forget about preservatives.

French fries can't be too far behind. Just slightly better due to the thickness of the potato. If frozen ones are used, you can be sure that it is dusted with preservatives, another word for pesticides.

Some of them contain some nutritional value, like nuts and or fruits, so are better than others that have nothing to offer, but they still have too many undesirable ingredients and thats why they have to be considered junk food. There are foods that are generally not considered junk food, but probably should be, including foods that contain sugar, other overly refined products and "excess" animal fat and even any fat.

Glaring examples are pancakes and french fries, Pizza, sausage, bacon and all denatured food, like white bread, pasta and rice. They may not contain as much junk, but their balance between nutrition and empty calories and/or excess fat, leaves them in that category. Any beverage with excess sugar should be avoided as well. I am sure there are many more that I am not even aware of.

Read the labels and make up your own mind if they have too much "junk" ingredients or not.

If you don't bring them home, chances are, you will eat less of them and avoid the fast food restaurants and probably most of the restaurants that are not considered "fast food" as well.

Put your shopping cart in high gear when crossing the bakery and keep your eyes straight ahead and don't pay attention to your ears that may be telling you that that pie or cake is calling your name. If you just have to have some cookies, consider some Kashi, soft baked ones or try to find something else that is not as bad as others.

GLUTEN

A substance found in wheat and some other grains. It is used to give body to many processed foods, besides bread, even ice cream and I suspect even margarine, etc. Although whole wheat is a very nutritional food, many people are gluten intolerant and unfortunately have to find ways to avoid it. The best way is to just avoid bread and other processed foods as much as possible.

PRESERVATIVES

Whether natural or chemical, makes food last longer. The bugs won't eat it, but us dummies will. You can be sure it is added to all processed foods, no matter where they are found, even in canned foods and frozen ones and fresh produce as well.

Even more stuff that our bodies have no idea how to deal with and it and just shoves it into our fat cells hoping to have time to figure it out later, but never does and compounds our health problems, including overweight.

FAST FOOD RESTAURANTS

I do like some of them and I feel sure that they contain a little bit of nutrition, but am pretty sure that they contain a lot more stuff that does not and anything you put in your mouth that is not nutritious is detrimental to your health.

A lot of them have side salads, but those dressings can be a killer and need to be eaten with caution, but most likely are still better than some other choices. Still I don't think an occasional Whopper will kill you.

I have no cravings for any of them and so just try to avoid them, but once in a while they are just convenient, so...........Any port in a storm!

We don't know everything that is a part of the ingredients, but the most obviously unhealthy ones are french fries, white, refined bread and sugary drinks and dont forget those nasty preservatives.

MSG

Monosodium glutamate. Everybody is allergic to this non essential amino acid, but it is added to many processed foods, including stuff found in restaurants, whether fast or slow and It improves taste and acts on your brain to make you crave more of it, similar to nicotine. It is rated as generally accepted as safe by the FDA, but still they are concerned about disclosure for some reason and I think it is because some people are highly allergic to it.

It is not only detrimental to your body's needs, but makes you want to overeat, causing obesity. The more whole foods you eat, the more satisfied you are and leaves you craving less food in general. It is the salt derived from glutamic acid and can be found naturally in many foods, but in much less concentrated forms than found in what is added to food. Chinese food (American) is prepared with a lot of it. When people claim that chinese food doesn't stay with them, I think that it is just because the MSG is leaving you wanting more. (Dont bother to ask for Chow mein in China, they will think you are nuts)

It is sold in the supermarket under the trade name Accent and a couple of others. Besides enhancing flavors, it can be used as a meat tenderizer and a replacement for some of your sodium chloride if you have to reduce your intake and don't want to do it any other way.

I think it should be avoided as much as possible.

IODINE

An essential chemical element to keep your Thyroid healthy and it affects several organs in your body. Most of our agricultural land is Iodine depleted, but it is found in seafood and dairy products, especially in yogurt, but also in eggs. Iodised table salt contains some and so does many multi-vitamins. Deficiencies can result in mental problems and other problems like breast cancer as well as other cancers and Goiters etc. Taking too much can also cause severe problems and some people have an allergic reaction to it, so dont go crazy. I don't know how much is too little or too much, but I think that if you consume dairy products on a regular basis and some seafood may be sufficient. Farmed fish may be classified as sea food, but doesn't come from the ocean and so has no Iodine unless added to their food, but how do you know?

Freshwater fish is also "Not" seafood and will have no iodine either, unless it runs through iodine rich soil. We have no idea, whether it does or not and I am not saying to not eat it, but be aware.

Dont think that just because you eat a lot of catfish, you are getting plenty of iodine.

If you take a multivitamin/mineral tablet once a day, make sure it contains Iodine unless you have specific reasons to avoid it.

STANDARD RESTAURANTS

They are in business to make money just like everybody else and do what they think they need to, to get your business.

They are usually not concerned with your health, but the intelligent ones put forth some effort into making the food taste good and your stay a pleasant one, but what is surprising to me is that many don't seem to put any effort into it at all, but they know that some people will just eat anything, anywhere and if they get enough patrons to satisfy them, that is all that they need. Many of them can easily be identified by the flavors of over seasoned food with undesirable additives.

Like most people, I like to eat out once in a while and have my favorite restaurants, but don't go there for my health, I just consider it a "Cheat day" and try to not be too stupid about it and spend the rest of my day trying to be a good little soldier.

Our destiny is in our own hands and we have to take responsibility for it.

REFINED FOOD

By now just about everybody that hasn't been living under a rock knows that overly processed foods like sugar, white bread, etc. don't even have to be digested and go straight into your bloodstream and spike your Glucose levels, which causes your body to pump out insulin at an alarming rate to turn it into body fat and may pump out too much and drive your blood Glucose too low and therefore causing you to be hungry and create a fat storing cycle.If it does get too low, it may even reduce your energy and you may not want to eat at all, putting you in danger of a hypoglycemic shock and it is especially detrimental to diabetics, but may also encourage others to become diabetic. There is no way to justify eating them. They are not healthy stuff to eat and I have avoided them for many years already. Having said that, if you are intent on eating some, just try to make good choices by reading labels. Not the Nutrition label, but the ingredients and if you think it has too much sugar, including some other words that they use to camouflage it, like high fructose syrup, etc.,or things that have names of stuff that you don't recognize, try to pick something else that is a better choice.

Food in restaurants don't have labels, so you just have to remember what is what.

Some of the Protein bars are probably ok, like Clif Builders, but some are not and again, They are certainly a better choice than your standard candy bar or apple pie.

Many Kashi cookies and cereals may be ok, but some don't taste so good, at least not as far as I am concerned.

When it comes to grain products like bread, pasta, rice, etc., they should only contain whole grains. Multi-grain bread just means that it has different grains in it, but not necessarily whole grains and brown bread may be artificially colored refined bread to fool you.

You won't find any labels in the bakery, so you have to just try to decide if it is something that you should be eating or not.

Refined sugar not only drives up your glucose level, turning what is not used for energy into fat, but it also eats away at teeth, being a big contributor to cavities, etc. It is also empty calories and has no nutritional value. It tastes good though and may be found in a multitude of processed foods as well as used to sweeten tea and coffee, etc.

Overly refined flour, has little nutritional value to offer and turns to paste without fiber and sticks to your intestines, where your body keeps trying to do something with it, poisoning your body and along with meat, which contains no fiber, can clog your intestines for years and cause polyps and maybe even cancerous ones.

It also diverts your energy that needs to be used for other chores to repair and maintain your body.

COFFEE/TEA ETC.

 I don't think a couple of cups a day is going to impair your health, but the fly in the ointment is the stuff you add to it, like sugar and artificial creamers. Artificial sweeteners have no calories, but fool your body into thinking that it does and will cause a rise in glucose and subsequent rise in insulin. There has been many studies lately that claim that it causes cancer and other ill effects as well.

I say, just avoid it. Its not as hard as you may think, we are creatures of habit. Give light coffee a try, ½ caffeinated and ½ decaf. I find it even tastier than regular coffee.

BOOZE

No matter what it is made from, it is yeast turning sugar into alcohol and it will spike your blood glucose levels. You may have heard that red wine is good for you, but it is Reserverol from the pigment of grapes that provides it and it is found in all red grapes, cranberries, etc. and doesn't need to have alcohol in it. Alcohol, if overly consumed can destroy your liver causing Cirrhosis. Remember that everything we consume has to be processed through our liver and if we destroy its effectiveness, we would cause our bodies to be in big trouble and shorten our lives.

Just because many of our movie heros spent their free time in bars, doesn't mean that we should.

FIBER

There are two different kinds of fiber, soluble and insoluble. Soluble fiber gets into your bloodstream and helps keep arteries from clogging up with stuff wanting to stick to their walls and causing heart attacks and strokes. Insoluble fiber is the one that helps to keep food moving in your intestines and helps to keep them clean. I think it does other good things for your body as well, but just remember that it is good for you.

SALT

We need a little in our diet, but most of us get way too much and it causes water retention and hardening of the arteries and high blood pressure, which could lead to heart problems, overweight and strokes.

All processed foods have some, so just be aware and avoid the salt shaker. If you think you can't live without it and need an easy fix, try "No salt", it is potassium chloride and tastes about the same as sodium chloride. You would never even notice any difference if you didn't already know what it was. It is the substance that is used in lethal injections, but harmless in a much lower concentration. You can also rotate it with the sodium chloride or mix them together. Try to use more black pepper, which is a strong anti-oxidant and you will get used to it and not crave the salt, or at least not so much. Cravings for salt is just like a craving for anything else, you can train your body to do without it.

Cayenne pepper is very beneficial to your health. Many people don't like it at all, but it is a developed habit and can be built up by using a little at a time and slowly building up your resistance to it.

Morton must have been reading my mind. I just found out that they now have a "Light salt" half sodium chloride and half potassium chloride. I tried it and it tastes great and I will never buy plain salt ever again. It can also be used for cooking and anything else you use regular salt for.

MSG can also be used, but I don't think that is a good choice.

CINNAMON, ETC.

A natural pesticide, don't get crazy with it, but it helps to balance your blood sugar, use capsules with added chromium, which also helps to lower LDL cholesterol (the bad one). Other natural seasonings are very beneficial as well for various reasons, but you have to know which ones make your food taste better to you and act accordingly. If you are interested, get a copy of "The vitamin bible" or even better "The worlds healthiest foods" or better yet.........both.

BUTTER/MARGARINE

This controversy has raged for many years, with both sides having some logic to support their argument. Butter is 100 % saturated animal fat, which is not heart healthy and when the facts first appeared in the 1950's, manufacturers scrambled to produce a product to replace it that looked and tasted similar and they came up with margarine, but they hydrogenated otherwise healthy oils to get the physical similarity and later was found to be even worse for our health, so the scientists found other ways to make the margarine that avoided the hydrogenated oil (trans fat) and it is usually found in tubs. Again you have to read the labels. Still its a processed food and we don't know exactly what they are doing to it, I suspect that they add Gluten, but I am not sure. Take your choice, butter, margarine, neither or moderation. I choose to use a little good quality margarine in moderation, but many nutritionists still disagree with that. However I don't think that they know either.

Fast food restaurants got slammed for using trans fats as well to cook their food, but many are making efforts to replace it with something else, not because they are concerned with your health, but worried that it could cause them to lose business.

A lot of other processed foods contain some and again, read the labels and watch out for those words that you don't recognize. Who knows what regular restaurants use, it seems to me that they haven't really been investigated yet and I doubt if they ever will be, but if you only eat out once in a while, I don't see any significant problem.

VEGETABLE OILS

More ongoing controversy. Many people claim that they destroy their benefits when cooked with at temperatures above their smoke point and they also spoil easily even if they don't appear so. there is other controversies, between one oil and another.

Others seem to disagree as they continue to recommend them for cooking. Coconut oil is 100 % saturated plant oil, but doesn't have the same detrimental effects as animal fat. It is reputed to have the highest smoke point of all the veggie oils and I have accepted that and that's all I use for cooking, except for occasional margarine when I am after that particular flavor, but I try to cook on low heat as much as possible, just in case. All fats and oils have over 100 calories per tablespoonful, but a negligible glycemic index.I keep my coconut oil in the fridge where it solidifies, so first I portion it off into tiny plastic containers and when I plan to use some, I take out a container to warm up. If its warm outside, I just stick it outside for a while to liquefy. With a little thought, I am sure you are smart enough to figure this out.

FAT

Since animal fat is mostly saturated, it can lead to heart disease if too much is consumed and therefore should be kept to a minimum. since all fat and oils have more than twice the amount of calories than protein or carbohydrates, none of it should be overeaten. Vegetable oils have a variety of essential fatty acids and are essential to good health and an excellent source is seeds and nuts. Flax seeds have the most fatty acids in general and walnuts contain the most Omega-3, which most of us don't get enough of. Omega-6 is important to our health as well, but is abundant in many foods.

Some of the vitamins are fat soluble, like A, D and E, which is another good reason to not try to eliminate all fat from your diet.

Fat cells are like bubble wrap and store more than pure fat, like water and things that your body doesn't know what to do with, saving them for later. Since humans eat a lot more junk than other animals, their fat cells get jammed up with toxins, including pesticides and other chemicals and other manufactured stuff that is not real food. It makes us overweight and unhealthy.

DETOXIFICATION

I think its a good idea to help our bodies dump some of these undesirable things out of our fat cells once in a while and the best way that I have found to do it, is to take a heaping tablespoonful of Epsom Salts mixed in a 20 ounce glass of water and drink it the first thing in the morning, before eating anything and your body will dump water out of your system to flush it out and along with it will be the stored toxins. As soon as it starts working, keep drinking plenty of water and fruit and/or veggie juice to keep it moving and replace some of the valuable nutrition that your body needs and if you don't, your body will try to reabsorb these toxins and poison your system. Pick a day that you don't have to go anyplace, just in case.

When somebody starves to death, it is actually, because the toxins that are being shed along with the water in the fat cells is being re absorbed in concentrated quantities and poisoning the body. This is also a primary reason to be sure to drink plenty of water and/or other liquids while losing weight.

Remember Gandhi's long term fasts? He didn't just stop eating, but went through a process of detoxifying his system, before eliminating food altogether. Don't bother to attempt this, its not necessary and could be very dangerous.

WATER

Reportedly, we can not survive more than 3 days without water, true or not, it is extremely important to our health. Our bodies need it for a host of activities, including washing toxins out of our body and we should drink water, whether thirsty or not, until our urine is clear, otherwise your body will try to re absorb undesirable substances. Digestion occurs all the way from the your mouth to your anus. Are you old enough to remember suppositories? Only highly refined food is absorbed directly from the stomach and starchy foods are absorbed shortly after, but most other substances are absorbed along the way and into the colon. The very reason that gay men are so susceptible to the HIV virus.

A controversy continues between distilled and mineral water. Distilled water helps to flush more toxins out of the body, but some complain that it also washes some vitamins and minerals out of the body. I don't consider it to be a big issue, because if you are eating a lot of healthy food, you are putting them right back in. I don't plan to lose any sleep over it.

Drinking plenty of water may help to prevent kidney stones and distilled water is probably better for that purpose.

Water has a zero glycemic index rating, but don't get the wrong idea that drinking a glass of water with a high glycemic food will balance it out, because it doesn't.

If your diet consists of fast foods and other junk food, you are not very interested in your health and longevity anyway. You are just committing "Unintentional suicide" or "Apathetic suicide".

SMOKING

While on the subject of suicide, everybody by now knows that this is a very serious No-no.

George Burns lived to be 100 and reportedly smoked 10 to 15 cigars a day, but he was an exception to the rule. Don't think you can get away with it.

The question in my mind is "Was he inhaling them? or just promoting his irresponsible image?" I started smoking in my youth when everybody already knew that it was not a healthy thing to do, because I thought it was being a grown up along with drinking alcohol and other forbidden things for kids to do.

Besides ruining your own health, it is pretty hard to convince your children not to smoke, when you yourself continue to smoke.

I don't know the statistics, but you can easily find information on famous entertainers, who died at a young age and even though some died from drug overdoses or heart attacks, many, many more died from smoke related illness. Some notable ones are Nat King Cole, Michael Landon, Victor French, Yul Brynner, etc.

LOW FAT MILK

Another healthy food that many people are intolerant to and they have to avoid it or buy a substitute like Lactated milk.

In fact people may be allergic to anything and if the doctor tells you to, you will have to take it upon yourself to try to eliminate that item from your diet.

For the rest of us, it is still fairly high in calories, 120 per 8 oz. but has a negligible glycemic index.

NUTS AND SEEDS

Packed with good nutrition including essential fatty acids and essential amino acids, but very high in calories. ¼ cup of any of them has over 200 calories, but a low glycemic index. This is due to the high oil content. Many are poisonous, so if you don't know for sure, just avoid eating them. There are plenty that we know are safe. Don't go picking wild stuff in the woods without the proper knowledge. They should be eaten raw or roasted, but be careful if they are salted, which improves their flavor. Take a handful and roll them around on a kitchen towel to get rid of some of it.

PROTEIN

This is a word that confused me for a long time, because it is used in a very irresponsible way as far as I am concerned.

Only animals contain protein, which are the building blocks that make up most things in their body, but proteins are made from different combinations of amino acids, which is the important thing for us to consider. Humans, being animals need these amino acids for it to build its own Protein. The scientists tell us that there is a yet unknown amount of them, but they have identified 23 that they consider essential, because we have to get them from food. Many others can be converted from other amino acids in our food.

NO plant food contains protein, regardless of what it says on that can of beans. That is what is loosely called incomplete proteins, because they have MANY of the essential amino acids in sufficient quantities, but only Quinoa and some sea weeds contain enough of all of them to be considered complete and still, to call them protein is a misnomer in my estimation and may bring you to the wrong conclusion when making food choices.

Most animal products contain all the essential amino acids, but since they have been used to make other protein, they have to be broken down, so that we can use them to build our own protein. Its like tearing down a brick building and then taking the bricks to build another one.

Therefore its easier and more expedient for us to get our amino acids from plants, since our bodies can just select them to build and repair our bodies. All plant food contains all the essential amino acids, but most in too little quantity to be really usefull. Its fine for deer and cows, because they eat an enormous quantity, grazing and walking all day long. Ever hear the expression "Eating like a horse"?

But to make it simple for us humans, any kind of beans and nuts contain most of them and any kind of grains contain the missing ones. they don't have to be eaten in the same meal, but many moons ago, somebody already figured this out and that is why rice and beans is a staple in many countries and beans and corn in others.The problem with this is that they always use white refined rice in their mix, but it tastes really good. Another thing I don't like is they don't vary their types of beans. In Puerto Rico they make red kidney beans with refined rice and sometimes use pinto beans and in Cuba they use black beans. Like all foods, they each have their own nutritional differences as well as flavor and I think its much better to vary them. Beans are not only too tough to eat raw, they are also toxic and they need to be cooked for a long time, which makes canned beans an acceptable alternative to dried. It also saves you electricity, time and wash up, etc. Many are even flavored, so they taste good all by themselves. Baked beans have too much sugar added to them.

BLOOD GLUCOSE SPIKING

Insulin is the product that is generated by the Pancreas to govern our blood glucose level and keep it under a certain level and some foods raise it more than others. It is best to prevent these spikes from occurring and negating the necessity for the insulin and the way to do it is to not eat food that cause it to spike or at least, moderate what we eat, by eating low glycemic foods along with the high glycemic ones.

Animal products don't in itself drive up glucose and neither does most plant food that is considered vegetables at the supermarket. The exceptions being root vegetables, except maybe for carrots, which contain a lot of fiber and take longer to process. Grains, especially if they are refined and many sweet fruits are considered too high in glycemic index. However I have read many books on the subject and none of them tell us how high is too high and almost all of them don't even tell us the Glycemic index of individual foods. The only book that I found that lists many of them is "The worlds healthiest foods". this is a big book and reasonably priced and has tons of information on different foods, including rating them for nutritional content and importance and I strongly advise everybody to get a copy of this book. Mine sits on the table in front of me and is my food bible for frequent reference. Besides eating food that spikes your blood sugar, if you take in more calories than you burn off, it will also be added to your body fat, so if you are worried about being overweight, it is pretty simple. Spiking your blood glucose causes immediate storing of fat and taking in too many calories does also. Oh, yes and going for a long time without eating causes your metabolism to slow down to conserve energy for the hibernation.

If you are diabetic and your blood sugar stays too high, it destroys your body, but taking medication to lower it, is detrimental to your liver. The best answer then, is in prevention and trying to not let it get too far out of range in the first place.

Again refined sugar and grains should not even be on your shopping list along with some other no-no foods, you know what they are.

High glycemic foods can be tempered by eating them along with low glycemic foods, like animal products and most vegetables, for example whole grain toast with eggs, meat and/or vegetables followed with some fruit, etc. Give it some serious thought and come up with your own combinations. This is especially important for diabetics.

Unfortunately apple pie and ice cream won't combine with anything no matter how much thought you put into it. Keep these types of food for very occasional cheats, if at all.

I would like to point out that the books that I have read only talk about potatoes and carrots, being root vegetables, but in many other places in the world they eat a multitude of other root veggies and are a great contributor to their diabetes.

VEGETABLES

As regarded by your local supermarket is generally highly nutritious in vitamins, minerals and fiber and smatterings of other stuff as well. they are all different in nutritional value, but all of them in general can be considered high on the nutritional list and low on the glycemic index and calories. Avocados are a little high in calories, but low on the glycemic index scale. Salad greens may appear very similar, but can be very different in composition. Spinach is higher rated in nutritional value than any other food and has about 40 calories per cup and a very low glycemic index and romaine lettuce is rated almost as high for nutritional value and also a low glycemic index, but only 8 calories per cup.

Never forget that variety is the name of the game.

Don't attempt to satisfy all your nutritional needs with a couple of foods. A meal consisting of meat, potatoes, vegetables and maybe a little fruit for dessert is a balanced meal, but don't eat the same thing everyday. I think even my mother knew that and we have animal instincts that guide us as well.

When you overeat foods that are not nutritionally combined or are just wrong foods, your body will protest and only remain satisfied for a short time. It may even cause you to feel nauseous.

MUSHROOMS

While on the subject of vegetables, mushrooms deserve special mention.

Years ago, there was a lot of buzz about Shiitake mushrooms, because somebody had discovered that they had antibacterial properties like garlic and vinegar do, but Crimini mushrooms are rated much higher on the nutritional scale and in fact they come in number 3 behind spinach and Swiss chard. I have never liked them and I don't know why, I think it is some kind of paranoia. Every time we went to a good restaurant that served sauteed mushrooms, my wife would order a side dish of them and then eat maybe one and I would eat most of the rest of them, not because I liked them, but I knew they were nutritious and I hate to waste money and I had to pay for them anyway. They have a round head and may be anything from a little button mushroom to a big portabella.

DARK CHOCOLATE

Very high in antioxidants and other nutritional value and is derived from the Carob plant, but it is bitter and is used in a lot of junk food and ruined with a lot of sugar.

There is no reason for it, because chocolate goes well with fruit and often is, but still the sugar needs to be avoided. Maybe somebody has figured a way, but I don't know what it is, if they have.

I tried adding some to my nutritional blender drink and it ruined the batch.

SWEET FRUITS

Any vegetable that contains seeds is technically rated as a fruit, but the unsweet ones are lumped in with the vegetables at the store. Sweet fruit is very nutritious and tasty, but always higher in calories and glycemic index, so their quantity should be limited, especially if you are worried about your weight or are diabetic. They can also be balanced with lower glycemic and lower calorie foods.

Many people recommend eating them by themselves and that may carry some merit, if you have special problems with digesting foods, but if you want to keep your blood glucose balanced, then you need to eat them together or afterwards. Fruits that have a low enough glycemic index would be ok to eat by themselves, but I haven't been able to find any information that can tell me how low is low enough and which ones are those. I am thinking 60 or less, but this is just a guestimate. Better to just eat them with other non sweet food.

GRAINS

Nutritious and high in many essential amino acids and they should only be whole grain, because when they are overly processed, they remove most of the nutrition, including fiber and drive up their Glycemic index. I dont understand why everybody in this country seems to be in love with highly refined stuff, especially rice, the whole grain rice tastes good, but takes longer to cook. I buy Uncle Bens parboiled whole grain rice (It has already been cooked to a certain degree and only takes 10 minutes to prepare) and it tastes great.

When Portugal was colonizing South Africa and started raising rice in their fertile land many of the natives depended on it for most of their diet and when they started refining and striping the rice of many of its nutrients, the natives started getting sick, where the Portuguese were not and they found that it was because they were getting other food as well that they had stored on their ships.

Only some animals eat raw grains, and they don't taste good to us and like raw turnip greens, need something done to them to get us to eat them and this is the problem. Who eats Oatmeal without adding something to it to sweeten it, etc.? You can buy whole wheat flour, which tastes great for breading meats or thickening gravies, Whether refined or not, pasta and bread are high in calories, so.........Corn is a little different and has been genetically altered so many times that it is making people sick if they don't have enough other food to make up the bulk of their diet.

I think it was the Ivory coast in the 1990s that depended on corn for the bulk of their diet and had some disastrous problems with their crops and the United states offered to give them a couple of ship loads of corn to help them out and the president declined, because he said we had already ruined the nutrition in our corn to make it taste and look better and it would ruin theirs as well as many people wouldn't refrain from planting it, just like they did in Mexico some years before.

Bread is one of our biggest culprits in this country, it is high in calories and most people eat way too much of it and it is reported that, because of genetic altering it is adding to the problem of our overweight problems. Consider this, two slices of toast with butter or margarine contains about 400 to 600 calories, even if it is whole grain, not to mention the junk that has been added to make it.

Not that many years ago, bread would only last a couple of days, before getting stale or developing mold. Now it will last for many weeks without changing appearance and most people are thrilled with it, but consider this - How much preservatives (pesticides) do they have to add to it to obtain that result? Many of us have become addicted to it and find it difficult to eat without it.

In many other countries, the people are smarter than we are and don't eat bread. I went to a huge restaurant in Thailand and the first thing you see when you walk in the front door is a large goldfish pond and close by is a table selling loaves of bread. A friend of mine was ordering food and they told him that they didn't serve bread, so he went back to the entrance to buy a loaf and took it back to his table and everybody started making fun of him as the bread was only to feed the fishes, not to say that it was good for them either.

The original invention of bread was not specifically for eating, but to hold meat with so that your hands don't get too greasy and then if you are still hungry, you could eat some to fill you up. It was especially handy for people like coal miners that had to take their lunch to work.

Back then the bread was healthier than it is today, especially in the United States, where we seem obsessed with over processing and genetically altering everything we eat. It is showing up in our rapidly increasing obesity ratings. I consider it a national cancer like drugs and tobacco and overindulgence in alcohol.

There is some question about the genetic altering of wheat, but there is not much we can do as individuals about that now. If you are willing to overlook that and know how to make your own bread, then you can still avoid some of the problems. You can buy whole wheat flour, which is all I buy and just make your own bread. You can also buy wheat germ and sprinkle it on other foods, like yogurt and add it to stuff like scrambled eggs, etc. and not even notice the difference. That's what I do, but I am sure you can find many other things to sprinkle it on if you are interested.

Even so, the grains are nutritious and if you can find a way to eat them without first ruining them, then go for it. I think the easiest way is to prepare rice and beans, using only whole grain rice and avoiding adding junk to the bean mixture.

Most people eat refined rice and will get a large serving of rice with a little beans. I, on the other hand am all about the beans and will take a little rice and a lot of beans. Whole grain pasta may be a good second choice, depending on what you add to it.

I often buy small Barilla microwave meals called Italian entrees and are found on the canned meats aisle, but I only buy the whole grain pasta with a tasty sauce. It makes a tiny snack/meal for a cost of 330 calories in a 9 Oz. serving.

This is the other problem with grains, whether refined or not, they are still high in calories and we tend to eat too much of them. If a tiny Barilla meal contains 330 calories, just imagine what a big plate of spaghetti and a basket full of garlic bread has. I love it but,...............shudder!

RED MEAT

There is no controversy here, red meat is considered the worst meat for our health and Americans are the biggest consumers on earth, bar none. Even so Reindeer is the most common meat eaten in Scandinavian countries and lamb is the favorite in many other countries. Cows are worshiped and not eaten in India, but used only for milk and roam free in the streets along with rats. Cows are outlawed in Cuba and beef can only be bought in restaurants for tourists and locals are not allowed in. Americans appear to be in love with beef, but I think it is a clear case of "Monkey see - monkey do" and should be added to the list of foodstuff to try to limit consumption. I do like a good steak once in a while, but if you don't spend the money for an expensive cut of meat, that has been grass fed, and has not been subjected to hormone shots, it is too tough, takes longer to cook it and is tasteless unless you use sauces to flavor it up or grind it up, so............Whats the point?

Veal is against the law in Thailand and foie gras (French method of force feeding ducks) is against the law in several countries and I think both of these things should be against the law in the U.S., due to the inhumane method of fattening animals. If we are going to insist on eating meat, they should be raised and slaughtered in the most humane method possible.

Horse meat is sold in butcher shops in France and other heavily french influenced countries like Morocco. Dog meat is sold in butcher shops in the Philippines, Indonesia, Malaysia and other countries with similar customs and I don't think you will find any stray cats in many poor countries.

ANTELOPE

Home, home on the range where the deer and the antelope roam, must have been written in Africa, as antelopes are not native to the United States, regardless of what many old westerns say about going out and killing one. Deer however is abundant and provides good quality protein.

PORK

Even though banned by Muslims and Jews alike and even some Christian bibles tells you on the first page to not eat cloven footed animals, it is surprisingly, the most common of all meat eaten in the world. I would have guessed chicken, but its not and only runs in second place. I have often wondered why we don't see more pork on menus and in supermarkets. ground pork only occupies the smallest of spaces in the supermarket, but to me a pork burger sandwich is at least as tasty as a beef burger and is much healthier and cheaper than the beef. If people were more familiar with it, it would revolutionize the burger joints. Thats ok, I will just continue making my own. A nice pork chop is delicious and more tender to eat, without having to spend a lot of money for it. It also makes a superior stew than beef. I am not an advocate of deep fried foods of any kind, but if you are going to eat them anyway, wouldn't it be nice to have the opportunity of having some deep fried pork for a change like what is sold in many other countries?

Ham is a food that contains way too much salt and is difficult nowadays to find any that even tastes good. Many years ago, we would go to the butcher shop and get some sliced boiled ham and it was so delicious, half of it wouldn't even find its way home, but those days are long gone along with that nice ham steak that you used to be able to get at a restaurant for dinner. I find meat of any kind from the Deli doesn't even taste like meat to me. I do eat some ham, but I only buy little packages of Oscar Meyer boiled ham and only use one or two thin slices on a whole wheat sandwich thin with one slice of cheese (also high in sodium). Bacon is on the not recommended nutritional list, but I like it and have a few slices once in a while with my breakfast or a couple of tiny BLT's.

CHICKEN

One of the most commonly eaten meat in the world. It is cheap, tender and delicious and can be cooked in a host of different ways and canned chicken breast makes a cheap and quick chicken salad and it doesn't have a lot of junk added to it. It is right near the top of my list of favorite foods.

SEAFOOD

The best protein you can eat, providing that it hasn't been ruined by humans.

In the seafood market, you can find fish as high as $40. a pound or more. "Fresh fish" laying on top of some ice, may come from Guatemala, where fishing boats may have been out for weeks and then processed and shipped to wholesalers, who keep it on ice and then turn around and sell it to fish markets where it lays around on ice until somebody buys it. Sometimes you buy it and it tastes great and sometimes it doesn't and you have just wasted your money, Farmed fish like Tilapia is cheaper and tastes great and if you are just after taste and basic nutrition, It does not contain the metal contamination found in wild fish and it is a good buy in my opinion. It may be missing Omega-3 and some other things, but they can be gotten from other foods or supplements. Be aware that Atlantic Salmon is farmed fish that color has been added to try to make it look more appealing and it is always from a foreign country where oversight may be lax. Large ocean fish usually have more metal and other contaminants than smaller or more moderate sized fish. I prefer to buy frozen fish. It is cheaper and tastes great. However, I bought some Tilapia and Mahi-mahi from Walmart and it was terrible and I won't get it again. It didn't even taste like the real thing and I suspect that Walmart may have been duped.

And by the way, the reports are that seafood is the number one food for not getting what you are paying for. It is difficult for even the experts to tell and sushi restaurants are reported to be the biggest culprits.

OTHER PROTEINS

Andrew Zimmern or Anthony Bourdain can tell you that almost any kind of animal will be eaten in some place around the world, including parts that would turn our stomachs to even think about eating.

THANKSGIVING

Originally it was raccoon that was served, not turkey and one was sent in a cage as a present for president Coolidge, an animal lover, who instead adopted it as one of his pets.He was not the only president to keep raccoons as pets. You could walk down the street and ask any person that you meet and they will tell you that raccoons carry rabies, but this is only parroting. All land mammals are susceptible to rabies and it is not just limited to raccoons. Remember "Old Yeller?" Its about a dog that got rabies from wounds from rabid wild hogs.

EGGS

The whites have all the essential amino acids and the yolks have a lot of other good stuff for you, most likely its cheaper than other things and easier to prepare, eat and digest. I think it is a great choice. I pledge to never throw away an egg yolk for any reason, I don't care what any professional cooks say.

LOW FAT MILK

Contains all the essential amino acids and good quantity of calcium, but some people are lactose intolerant and have to avoid it. Yogurt, cheese and any other thing containing milk has the same advantages and disadvantages and cheese usually contains more salt than ham does (At least the cheap processed cheese does) There is real cheese and processed cheese, so...........I don't know about the ingredients of real cheese, I can't afford it.

SO, I WANT SOME ANIMAL PROTEIN FOR SUPPER, WHICH ONE SHOULD I EAT?

All animal products will have all the essential amino acids, but they also have other stuff to offer, so just like other food, we should eat a variety. If you have to think about it, why select the one that offers the least benefits to your health or that cost the most or consumes the most time and energy to prepare? Treat yourself nice, but not foolishly.

So now we know what food is good to eat and what is not and now all we have to do is put it all together into an eating plan.

At the end of the day, what I am after is something that tastes good to me and gives me the excellent nutrition that I am looking for and at the lowest possible price without sacrificing either.

Yes! I want it all and after chasing rainbows I am finally finding the answers I have been looking for. It is actually very simple, but many of us have not stopped long enough to recognize it. The flood of the power of suggestion has carried us downstream and we have lost sight of the basic truth. During the TV commercials, click mute and give it some thought. We dont need to be sheep, we have more brain power than that and need to exercise it. While driving, don't take your eyes off of the road, but use that as a time to give some thought to your eating habits as well.

FRUIT/VEGGIE JUICERS

Muscle man, Jack La lanne made these popular in the 1960's and it became a big money maker and a nutritional movement, people ran like Gazelles to get one, so that they too could be a healthy, muscle man, but people forget that he was a muscle man long before these juicers were even invented and he was making money to promote them.

He was also a muscle man, before the Big Mac was invented and if push came to shove, the veggie juice would win hands down. Having said that, I don't like them at all for three main reasons-

They remove the fiber and other nutrition associated with it and four fifths ends up in the trash, wasting a lot of nutrition and money. Juice with fiber removed has about 2 or 3 times the calories and a higher GI load.

I have a much better plan and will tell you shortly. Chew on your fingernails until I get to it.

FOOD COMBINING BOOKS

These are all about not eating protein in the same meal with starches, because your body has to produce conflicting chemicals to break them down and it hampers digestion.

When you eat protein, your body pumps out hydrochloric acid to break it down and when you eat starchy foods, including root vegetables, grains and maybe very sweet fruits, you body has to provide a conflicting chemical to process them and the two things oppose each other and hamper the digestive process. It is probably not a big deal for most of us, but still it could be a healthier way to eat, except for one glaring problem that they overlook.....eating starches or very sweet fruits by themselves will spike your blood sugar.

The hero then is vegetables, including non sweet fruits, because they don't take much of anything to digest and can be eaten with anything, so......................

you can have a non protein meal like a baked potato with a serving or two of any kind of vegetables or a tomato sandwich, etc.

If you want to eat a protein meal, you can eat any kind of animal products along with that same choice of vegetables and avoid the starch in the same meal, like with a sandwich made with meat or any other combination of meat and starches. There is not much chance that you will be eating much meat with very sweet fruits.

NUTRITION AND WEIGHT CONTROL SIMPLIFIED—PART TWO

THE BASIC IDEA OF THIS PLAN

To avoid blood sugar spikes, in order to avoid the necessity of needing excess insulin and to prevent high blood glucose from being immediately stored as fat, to shrink our stomachs and intestines, which has a great effect on lowering our hunger and to keep our metabolism running at full throttle. At the same time to lower our calorie intake and keep our blood sugar within a reasonable moderate range and to allow our body to seek a normal body weight. so.................

The way to do this is to eat tiny, frequent (2 to 4 hours apart), well balanced snacks throughout the day, instead of eating big meals that also cause blood sugar spikes and more fat storage and of course, a tougher job for our bodies to deal with.

Eating a tiny snack/meal more often than the usual 3 times a day will keep your metabolism on its toes, so it doesn't get the idea that you are starving and slow down to conserve the fat stores that you may want to get rid of.

You know what the principal combinations of food are and you can make up your own creations based on your likes and dislikes. Foods that have a high glycemic index, need to be combined with food that have a low glycemic index to balance out their effect on your blood glucose. All junk food needs to be avoided as much as possible and if you are trying to lose weight, you need to give some thought to the calorie content.

If you are trying to lose weight, it only takes a little thought to find ways to trim the calories without sacrificing your nutrition or having to never eat some foods that you like, not just the ones that have become habit.

Nuts and seeds are very nutritious food, but one cup may be over a thousand calories, but just a few a day gives you the nutrition that you are after without all the calories.

The only real foods that have a high glycemic index is root vegetables, (except for carrots), grains and sweet fruits. Animal products, nuts/seeds, fats and other vegetables do not. Keep in mind that variety is the name of the game and all grains should be of whole grain content and its best to eat all fruits and vegetables (Except the obvious ones, pineapple, avocado, etc.), especially root vegetables with the skin as thats is where much of the nutritional value is found as well as fiber and it lowers the average calorie count per volume and the glycemic index. The problem here is pesticides, so scrub them with a brass wire brush and cut away the bad stuff and whenever you can afford it, organic food is a better choice.

Most processed foods should be locked away and the key discarded, but there is a few that may be ok and some that can be occasionally eaten.

Both labels and careful thoughts have to be part of this equation and they should be kept to a minimum. Don't get into a panic, it took you a long time to put on that weight and poison your body and a slow reduction is the best course, you don't want your body to get the idea that you are the enemy and fight against you.

Forget about wasting money on magic bullets and quick loss schemes.

Forget about the scale, you already know if you are overweight or underweight and the scale won't tell you what to do about it. If you are doing the best that you can, that is all you can do and what the scale says, will make no difference. When you go to the doctor, he will weigh you to see if your weight indicates some other medical problem and you will have to depend on him/her to find a solution.

WHAT TO EXPECT

After a week or so, you will suddenly realize that your stomach has shrunk. Our stomachs, about the size of a grapefruit are actually found under our rib cages, with other vital organs, but you will begin to feel the difference in your belly (Often mistakenly referred to as your stomach) I can only assume that our intestines that is found curled up there has shrunk as well. Next you will be amazed to find that your cravings for junk food has subsided. Any desire you have to eat them is only habit, remembering that you like them, but it won't be a craving and just tell it to go away and don't come back another day or at least visit much less often. Besides bad habits and boredom, you will realize that four principal things cause us to overeat.

1   Not getting the nutrition that our body needs.

2   Monosodium glutamate and other addictive junk that makes us want to eat more.

3   Our stomachs and intestines being stretched out of shape and wanting to fill up the empty space.

4   Unbalanced blood sugar.

If you eat a small, calculated snack/meal and still feel hungry, wait for 20 minutes and if it doesn't subside, eat another one, etc.

You will slowly begin noticing obvious improvements in your health and you can be sure that your body is taking this opportunity to improve things that are not so evident as well as helping to prevent or slow down some upcoming problems.

After some time, you may find that lost color is returning to your hair and that your sex life is rapidly improving, your mind is becoming clearer and you are feeling terrific.

In fact you may be discovering that 16 year old that is still hiding inside of you, but being smothered under unhealthy tissue.

You are sure to stumble like on any plan, but that doesn't mean to give up. Just dust yourself off and get back on the horse. The less you cheat, the better off you will be. Some is always better than none, so never ever throw in the towel.

By eating in this much more nutritious manner, you may find toxins trying to escape through your skin, causing some eruptions, but with time, they will go away.

If you have a history of eating a lot of fiber depleted foods like animal products and denatured processed foods, you may have a buildup of toxins in your intestines and this plan will increase your fiber intake and slowly break this substance loose and push it down your intestinal tract and may cause some constipation, but will slowly straighten itself out. This would be a good time to think about cleansing by occasionally taking some Epsom salts.

20 years ago, freckling on my ankles was first pointed out to me, It is an indication of diabetes, but now, they are slowly clearing up and are much less freckled than they were those many years ago. Along with my doctor, I have been reducing the amount of medication that I take and hope to eventually end all of it, the only thing that may prevent it is any permanent damage I have done to my body.

TRYING TO LOSE WEIGHT?

A 300 calorie snack/meal every two hours is only 1800 calories per 12 hours.

400 calories every 3 hours is 1600 calories.

600 calories every 4 hours is 1800 calories and keeps your metabolism on its tippy toes.

If you have a snack meal of 300 calories, wait two hours to eat something else and if you eat 400 calories, wait 3 hours to eat something else and if you eat 600 calories, wait 4 hours, etc. In between, drink a nutritional blender drink if you like or a big glass of water.

A 20 oz. nutritional blender drink every hour takes 16 hours to make sure you get enough calories. You would have to be a fanatic to drink that much, but balance it out with a few other selections and you have a powerhouse weight reduction plan.

Besides that, try to limit bread and corn as much as possible.

Try this - Only drink nutritional drinks in the morning until noon if you don't work at a strenuous job and need more protein.

If you have been fasting overnight for many hours, your stomach and intestines will have shrunk a bit and you probably are not that hungry, but are just in the habit of eating that big breakfast and also you just have a taste for it, but guess what? you can still have that breakfast, but later on, by replacing another meal later in the day with it.

You can also tone it down. First thing in the morning, have two or three eggs with a nutritional drink.

3 boiled eggs with a nutritional drink is only about 300 calories and then go back to drinking just the nutritional drink as frequently as you want, until you feel you just have to have something else. Fried or scrambled eggs, instead will only add about another 100 calories or so. Avoid the toast, the potatoes, the grits and don't even think about eating pancakes, which is really sweet bread and then you want to put butter and sugary syrup on it…Really?….Shudder!

Pancakes and waffles taste good, but guess what? They should be on the same list with candy bars and apple pie. Who was it that decided that this would be something good to eat for breakfast? Fat albert?

WE ARE CREATURES OF HABIT

They can be changed with just a little bit of effort. Even though I knew it was a stupid thing to do, I smoked for 25 years and thought it was impossible to quit, but I kept running into other people that had and it finally sank in, that if they could do it, I could too and I did and now wonder why I ever smoked. For a few years, I always put milk and sugar in my coffee, but finally gave that up for unflavored coffee and now I have also changed to half decaf coffee and have just made it a habit that I don't even think about any more.

WHEN TO EAT

You need to eat something shortly after awakening, that is why it is called break fast. contrary to common belief, it doesn't have to be a huge meal, it depends on your activity level, but you want to eat something to let your body know you are not hibernating.

Dr Oz has hyped many times about eating that big breakfast, but he himself drinks a nutritional blender drink first thing in the morning, but doesn't bother to mention the ingredients or the philosophy of it, because it won't produce any profit. His wife Lisa is a vegan and makes the drinks for him. You can be sure it doesn't contain any animal products.

You dont want to eat close to bedtime, because your body needs to get heavy digestion out of the way, so that your body can concentrate on other functions it needs to perform while sleeping.

If you eat right before bedtime, your body has to spend that valuable time digesting food, instead of attending to other chores. "Don't eat after 8 PM" is an oversimplification. What if you are working shift work? What if you retire early? What if you take an afternoon nap?

food doesn't digest as well when you are lying down. Some foods are harder to digest and may cause acid reflux. Don't be a sheep, think for yourself, it can be fun and give you a sense of accomplishment, like it has done for me.

VEGANS SEEM TO FARE BETTER THAN MEAT EATERS IF THOUGHT IS GIVEN TO THE COMBINATIONS OF FOODS AND IF IT SATISFIES YOUR HUNGER.

Vegetables are always lower in calories and Glycemic Index, so can basically be eaten in unlimited quantities. Sorry apple pie is not a vegetable and neither is a snickers bar.

I don't think anybody has an urge to overeat vegetables, even if they are a Vegan. Another thing to consider is that consuming a lot of whole plant food will allow a much lower intake of toxins and a much higher intake of fiber.

Inhumane treatment of animals is a strong incentive to avoid eating animal foods as well. Some claim that the carbon dioxide produced by animal flatulence is destroying the ozone layer and plants produce oxygen. Cows are supposedly the biggest problem. Humans also produce flatulence as part of our normal digestive process. We may not be inclined to eliminate humans, but I think that eventually, eating a diet mainly of vegetables and avoiding the refined foods and meat with antibiotics and other stuff that may be injected into it, would calm this down and it is in effect, right in line with the food combining diet that is mentioned in some books for easier digestion by avoiding foods that fight each other by causing your body to pump out different chemicals to break them down and leaving more of your bodies energy to turn its attention to other bodily needs. Vitamin B12 needs to be gotten from animal products or from a supplement.

SUPPLEMENTS

There is some controversy here, but I take a multivitamin once a day, just in case. I think of multivitamins like stucco, you can not build a brick wall with stucco alone, but it helps a lot to fill in the missing chinks and gaps and multivitamins does the same thing to our bodies.

I also take a krill or fish oil supplement with Omega-3 and a couple of cinnamon capsules with chromium added and a COQ10 supplement. I don't get much sun so I take a vitamin D-3.

I also take a glucosamine tablet to lubricate my bone joints and help keep them from wearing out.

We also have to follow the doctors prescriptions and take whatever he/she thinks we need. I have found a decreased need for some medications, by following this eating plan, but talk it over with the Doc., you may not have the expertise to go it on your own.

HERE IS A LIST OF SOME OF MY SELECTED SNACKS/MEALS

Nutritional Blender Drinks

This is the backbone of my plan and is simple to make and will be delicious if made to my standard, or give it some thought, If you think you have a better idea, go for it.

Always keep in mind that variety is essential to good health.

Blend greens in a blender with filtered water and with or without a little fruit. I have a powerful blender, so I can blend anything that

I want to, but if you just use a standard blender, you can still blend any kind of greens, no not cabbage and don't try to get clever and add other nutritional stuff as it will throw off the flavor. Some of the veggies may be blended, but need to be steamed first, including broccoli, cauliflower, carrots, cabbage, etc. Start off slow so as to not discourage yourself and then do your own experiments if you like.

I spent more than a year doing a host of experiments and ended up back at square one. The easiest fruit to blend in a standard blender is bananas, tomatoes and any kind of berries, except cranberries. Other fruits may be easily blended, but the skins and seeds need to be removed first. I don't bother to blend the fruits that I enjoy eating. The greens that come with the strawberries are even more nutritious than the fruit, but they are not tasty. If you throw them into the blender with the berries intact, they disappear into the mix. I make a batch every couple of days and repackage it into recycled plastic bottles and store them in the fridge. Because of the very low calorie content and a negligible glycemic index, they can be consumed by themselves or with a higher glycemic food to neutralize it, but in fact they can be consumed with anything. They are very nutritious and you can consume as much as you like, because they keep your blood sugar balanced for a low price of calories and glycemic index.

Some greens have a harsher flavor than others, (that doesn't mean that they are not nutritious) so If they need a little help with the flavor, you can add a little store bought juice that doesn't have any added sugar. I found that V8- fusion, Ocean spray 100 % juice, Northland and Juicy juice get the job done very nicely or add more fresh fruit if you like. I try to use as much Organic ingredients as possible in my mix, Organic greens are not very expensive.

You can figure on an average of 100 calories per 20 oz. glass.

This delicious, nutritious drink can be consumed as often as you like and can even be your total food intake, at least for a long, long time. It beats the hell out of eating fast food and other junk food.

I may regret even suggesting this, because I don't think its a very good idea, but if you are going to eat some junk food anyway, you can at least tone it down by having a blender drink with it.

Some people call these blender drinks a "Green smoothie" and claim that is all you need to nourish your body and right or wrong, I don't like that idea. Hopefully we don't graze all day and I don't think we even could, so for that reason, I don't believe that we get enough essential amino acids and some other nourishment for our needs. Besides that, since we are blending our veggies, we are not doing the chewing that other animals do and may be detrimental to the health of our teeth and gums.

We couldn"t possibly eat enough salad to get the job done either and we won't even eat it without adding some nasty stuff to it.

V8 Juice

Even though the blender drinks are delicious and nutritious, this is a good alternative for a change of pace, it has only 50 calories per 8 oz. and very low GI. Buy the bottles, the cans have a foul taste, like all beverages. Be aware that it is a processed food and not as nutritious as fresh plant food, but it still beats the hell out of a sugary drink.

Peanut Butter Sandwich

Possibly my favorite snack/meal. Crunchy is lower glycemic and more nutritious than smooth and I think it tastes better.

1 whole wheat sandwich thin with one tablespoon of peanut butter and one spoonful of polaner all fruit is about 230 calories. The Polaner has no added sugar and is sweetened with fruit juice, it is only 30 calories per tablespoon. This makes a nutritious and delicious little sandwich and is very satisfying, add 8 oz of milk for another 120 calories. Read the label, for some reason some of them have added sugar. There is no need for it and the only ones that I found with sugar is the ones sold at Costco.

Micro-In Bag-Veggies

High on the nutritional list, including fiber. A 12 oz. bag of Broccoli/cauliflower/carrots contains only about 100 calories. Microwaving destroys a lot of the vitamins, but I eat about 2 bags of this a week. If you are not as lazy as I am, you can steam them.

3 minutes in the micro after piercing the bag a couple of times and let them sit for a few minutes to cool off and pour them into a large plate and sprinkle lightly with sea salt or "No salt" Potassium chloride, which tastes about the same or "lite salt", which tastes even better. There are also other vegetables that can be steamed as well, but I am not a cook and don't know a lot about it, but that doesn't mean that you can't be and you can add other seasonings if you like, but avoid overdoing anything with sugar and/or fats.

After a couple of weeks, I got weary of eating a whole bag and cut it in half. Eating just half and maybe adding some fruit or a boiled egg or two, etc. Leaving the other half in the fridge and the next day giving it one minute in the micro and doing the same thing again. Come up with your own plan. I have recently tried to micro them first and then add them to a blender mix with the greens and an orange or two and it came out with a terrific flavor, but no matter what a mix tastes like, I have gotten in the habit of adding a little store bought juice to improve the flavor to suit my tastes. You can do your own experiments and come up with something that you like. If you try to just drink something that doesn't taste good to you, you will quickly tire of it and go back to worse habits. It is quite possible to make a nourishing drink and also tastes terrific.

No matter what else I eat, I like to drink 4 or 5 of these 20 Oz. drinks over the course of a day.

You can even make some nourishing savory mixes for a puree type soup. If you are using a standard blender, you can cook the food first and then put it in the blender and if you have a powerful blender, you can blend everything and then just heat it up in the micro or on the stove.

I don't know enough about spices or I definitely would make some soup and put it in the fridge in recycled plastic bottles and just take out a cup or glass full once in a while, heat it in the micro and have a nice hot and nourishing drink, maybe instead of a coffee or tea, especially on a cold day. Never forget that you are the captain of your ship and the ultimate responsibility lies with you.

Bell Peppers

High on the nutritional list. Only 25 calories each. I chop them up and save them for munching on while watching TV. You can also have an egg or fruit or in fact anything you like with them. Some people prefer to use them for cooking.

Tomatoes

Even higher on the nutritional scale than bell peppers and one cup has 35 calories and a GI of 15.

If you can find fresh ones, picked at maximum ripeness, they are delicious and are a great snack all by themselves, but at the supermarket, this is a much bigger chore and only campari and grape tomatoes are very tasty to me. Still, any tomato can add nutrition to any sandwich along with some salad and at the same time cut down on the calorie and GI of the snack/meal.

Asparagus

Higher on the nutritional list than Broccoli. 43 calories per cup full and a GI of 15. Remove the tough ends and put them on a pan in the toaster oven for 12 minutes and give them a sprinkle of sea lite salt or NO-salt. I eat a whole pound of roasted asparagus for a snack/meal and it is very satisfying with only about 100 calories and the low GI. One of my favorite diet foods.

I save the tough ends and throw them in my high powered blender mix.

Baked Potato

Plenty of nutrition, but high in calories and glycemic index, so I don't eat it so often, but when I do I add a little margarine and some veggies and/or meat to tone down the GI. Some cut green beans combine well with it., balancing out the calorie per quantity and the GI.

Glass Of Low Fat Milk

By itself or with a cup or two of fruit or a small sandwich on whole grain bread or maybe an egg or two. About 120 calories for 8 oz. and lots of calcium, a negligible glycemic index. I buy Atkins dark chocolate nutritional drink with a screw top and just add enough to a glass to give it a robust chocolate flavor and save the rest in the fridge for next time.

Eggs

One regular size egg contains about 65 calories, zero glycemic index and lots of nutrition, protein and other stuff as well, but no fiber, like all animal products. It can be combined with anything you like. Some people still worry about the cholesterol content, but its a tiny amount and not as important as saturated animal fat, which your body uses to make excess cholesterol.

Breakfast Idea

One boiled egg, one banana and a nutritional drink or small glass of low fat milk or glass of fresh juice.

Low Fat Greek Yogurt

Get any one that has the fruit on the bottom and don't mix it up, that's where all the sugar is at.

Take a small spoon and just reach down to the bottom to get a little taste and when the yogurt is finished, just throw the rest of the preserves into the trash, you have no further need for it or buy plain yogurt and mix a little polaner fruit spread with it, if you don't like it plain.

Whole Wheat Sandwich Thins

A little controversial, but only 100 calories each and provides an easy way to get some protein, by making tiny sandwiches with egg salad, chicken salad, peanut butter, a slice of ham and/or cheese, tuna salad, etc.

Cheese and sandwich meats are a little high in salt and peanut butter contains some undesirable products, so don't overdo it. Mayonnaise has 90 calories per tablespoon.

Canned Tuna

Another of my favorites. Packed in water, a 5 oz. can only has 100 calories. zero glycemic index and makes a very cheap and nutritious snack/meal.

Tuna salad on two sandwich thins with mayo and a slice of tomato and a piece of lettuce cost less than 400 calories and is an excellent source of low fat protein. I usually find these on sale for about $1. a can and stock up. That's about $3.25 a pound as opposed to $40. a pound for fresh tuna that may or may not be fresh............. Really?

A Cup Of Cereal

Any kind that has little to no sugar or other junk added, with low fat milk.

You can add some chopped up fruit and/or nuts if you like. This is a little controversial also, so be your own judge. You are the captain of your ship. Read the labels.

Barilla Italian Entrees

Vegetable Marinara whole grain fusilli (9 Oz.) Micro for one minute. 330 calories.

Nutritional Bars

Some are great and some are not, but I especially like the "Clif BUILDERS" bar. They are delicious and I can not see any ingredients in this snack that is not good food. They contain a lot of Organic foods, 20 grams of essential amino acids and some vitamins at a cost of 270 calories per bar. I like the chocolate/peanut butter one the best, but everybody has their own taste buds. They are heavy, so you dont have to eat the whole bar at one time, you can just take a bite and leave the rest for later. (Ha-ha), that is only if you are stronger than I am. You might have better luck to select the one you like the least.

They are also low glycemic. I think the "Kind" bars are pretty good as well and they are low glycemic. I also like Kashi, soft baked cookies and one or two with a cup of plain coffee makes a good snack. My problem is that I like them too much and have a strong tendency to overeat them, so I just don't buy them so often.

Mashed Potatoes

If you have a real hankering for some, try making it with half potato and half cauliflower. In fact you can temper it with any veggie that you like. I like to add a can of cut green beans to mine. This goes for baked or boiled potatoes as well. Please leave the skins on.

I dont see any point to adding sour cream and even though potatoes taste better with butter or margarine, they don't taste disgusting if eaten plain with just a sprinkle of black pepper.

Pickles

Always a good snack choice if you like them. A little high on salt.

Jerky

Whether beef or turkey, can be a good healthy snack food if you like it.

A Handful Of Nuts And/Or Seeds

Raw or roasted, about 300-400 calories and Low glycemic.

If you are trying to lose some weight, keep them down to a smaller amount and eat them less frequently.

Can Of Beans

 Any kind, rotate them, about 300 calories. Has most of the essential amino acids in sufficient quantity and a host of other good nutrition. Very moderate glycemic index.

Strain them and throw away the juice, thats where most of the junk is. Don't rinse them or you lose too much flavor and I like to add some crushed red pepper to mine to spruce it up and increase the nutritional value or rinse them and add your own seasonings that you like.

Sardines

Very nutritious with lots of calcium since the bones are soft and eaten. Most of the calories is in the oil it is packed in, but I assume that you won't drink it. Still this oil is nutritious and beneficial to lower LDL cholesterol. You can also buy them packed in tomato sauce or even just water.

HERE IS AN IDEA FOR YOU

In between your meal/snacks you feel like consuming something, but you know you are not actually hungry, so how about drinking a big glass of water?

If you drink a big glass full and still are not satisfied, then go ahead and have something else.

RECIPES

Everywhere you look, you will find oodles of them, but I don't like them for a few reasons. They are all too complicated and waste too many ingredients, many that I have never even heard of, but even if they are terrific for the writers taste buds, I may not like it and will have wasted more time and money that I am not willing to part with.

Restaurants have no excuse to turn out crappy food, but somehow most of them manage to and thats all they do for a living. Another thing is that they are seldom considering nutrition, but merely taste. I want both and its possible. That doesn't mean I never have the urge to cheat and I do, but try to keep it from getting the best of me.

COMPROMISE

iF you were raised in Northern Thailand, you may be used to living on Dung beetles and if you came from different parts of Africa, you may have a taste for caterpillars, in the Philippines, Balut (duck embryos, eaten in the egg shell). but westerners have already developed their own taste buds and paranoias, so its important for each of us to learn to compromise healthy food with some not so good food that we enjoy in order to keep us satisfied, otherwise we will just give up and go back to worse habits. Remember that it doesn't have to be "All or nothing". just keep doing your best and it will get easier and easier, until it just becomes a habit.

ENHANCED PLAN

We know what is good to eat and how to balance our blood sugar and avoid food that is used to produce excess cholesterol, how to avoid some hidden no-nos, but it might be wise to think about lowering our digestive issues by avoiding foods that fight in the same meal, namely proteins and starches and very sweet fruits. It seems contrary to our plan, but there is no reason why they can't be combined. Here is some suggestions of how to do this -

Vegetable Sandwich

My mother used to eat a lot of onion sandwiches, sliced onions on buttered bread. I thought it was disgusting, even though I had never even tried it, but if you like it. go for it, but please use whole grain bread, even though it may contain too many undesirable ingredients, its still better than white, denatured bread. A tomato sandwich is maybe a better choice and you may have some ideas of your own. Have a big glass of nutritional drink with it and improve your little meal.

Whole Grain Pasta

With a non meat containing sauce. Keep it small and have a nutritional drink with it.

Meat With Vegetables

Without root veggies or grains.

Rice And Beans

no meat and no bread or other grains.

Salad With Chopped Boiled Eggs On It Or Other Animal Products

No grains or root veggies.

Eggs And Low Fat Ham

No bread and no potatoes.

Any of these things can be eaten with with unlimited veggies, except root veggies. you can also have a piece or two of fruit and unlimited nutritional drinks.

Steak and potatoes may be balanced as far as your blood sugar is concerned, but has no place on this plan.

EXERCISE

I am over 70, retired and have arthritis in my lower back and can't do a lot anymore and am pretty much of a couch potato, But still I invented a little routine with a 10 lb barbell and do them daily sitting in my big chair and have taken to wearing ankle weights most of the day and do a little leg exercise with them.

I also have an exercise ball that I sit on occasionally and just wriggling around on it, will tone up your innards.

With a little thought you can easily figure out how to get some of your muscles to stretch and move. Just keep doing something as much as possible, don't just lay around on the couch.

If you have a place to swim, that is a great way for a lazy person to get some exercise.

Get a hand exercise squeeze ball and play with it while watching the boob tube.

Walking and/or very light jogging is great exercise and you should try to get some in every day.

I have nothing against moderate exercise, it helps to tone you up and burns a few extra calories, but I will leave that up to you to make decisions based on your capabilities and desires. If you want to compete with Arnold, there are plenty of books out there to help you.

This may be the most important thing you have ever read and I consider that I have finally found the Holy grail. I hope that you have found this plan helpful and improves your life.

If this information has helped you in any way to improve your health, please pass it on to others so that they have the opportunity to improve their health as well, without having to pull their hair out and running around wasting time and money chasing rainbows. Lets make it a national effort to stamp out the money mongers and make our country a healthier one.

I toast your good health with a glass of nutritional drink.....
XOXO

SOME RANDOM THOUGHTS

A few years ago I was sitting in a chair getting a Pedicure and the lady next to me told me that she was a good cook. She was an older, overweight woman, who didn't look to be in the best of health and got me to thinking. "What does that mean?" Someone that makes appetizing food or makes healthy food? I think we all know the answer to that.

Most grocery stores have a health food section and it makes me wonder again "Isn't all food supposed to be healthy?" I guess not! The aisle with junk food is much larger and so is the bakery section, loaded with more junk food.

Get a sandwich at the Deli and they always ask if you want white bread or wheat bread? Isn't it all wheat bread? One white and one colored up to make it look healthier? Maybe some deep fried chicken is a better choice, well it sure tastes good. Its not their fault though, they are trying to make money by offering what we want to waste our money on, not to mention our health.

Cheers!

www.ingramcontent.com/pod-product-compliance
Lightning Source LLC
Chambersburg PA
CBHW030523290526
45786CB00004B/1592